Regina Benecke

360° feedback for therapeutic practices

Regina Benecke

360° feedback for therapeutic practices

Guidelines for introducing 360° feedback in therapeutic practices to increase cost-effectiveness

ScienciaScripts

Imprint

Cover image: www.ingimage.com

This book is a translation from the original published under ISBN 978-3-330-51417-1.

Publisher:
Sciencia Scripts
is a trademark of
Dodo Books Indian Ocean Ltd. and OmniScriptum S.R.L publishing group

120 High Road, East Finchley, London, N2 9ED, United Kingdom
Str. Armeneasca 28/1, office 1, Chisinau MD-2012, Republic of Moldova, Europe
Managing Directors: Ieva Konstantinova, Victoria Ursu
info@omniscriptum.com

Printed at: see last page
ISBN: 978-620-2-37529-0

Foreword

Employee assessment has a long tradition in business. However, the healthcare professions find this difficult, even though much has already been achieved in this area due to certification requirements and the associated quality assurance measures. However, unlike in the business world, appraisals rarely have any influence on salary increases. This book shows that therapeutic practices can also benefit from 360° feedback. Acting economically has long been a reality in the healthcare sector. Although many practices issue general satisfaction questionnaires to patients, therapists themselves are rarely evaluated. Until now, there has been no tool for this purpose. This book not only explains the importance of feedback, but also presents an evaluation tool for patients to assess the therapy and the therapist.

Regina Benecke

Occupational therapist, B.Sc.

Table of contents

CHAPTER 1

Introduction

Therapeutic practices are increasingly facing a variety of challenges. There are many reasons for this. For example, our society is changing from generation to generation. The much-cited demographic change is likely to lead to an increase in services in the health sector, but also to a shortage of skilled workers in this area. Werther (2015, p. 35) also describes the tense situation on the labour market. This makes it all the more important not only to select the right employees, but also to keep them satisfied, make the best possible use of their resources and provide them with ongoing training. 360° feedback is an analysis and evaluation tool that can be helpful in this regard. Comprehensive feedback on the behaviour, skills and competencies of employees can be obtained by evaluating their performance from the perspectives of their superiors, peers and customers.

Originally, 360° feedback was used to evaluate managers. However, Werther (2015, p. 18) also formulates it for employees. According to Werther (2015, p. 34f), feedback gives employees both appreciation, which can be a source of motivation, and the opportunity to participate in the development of the company. "Ultimately, participation also plays an increasingly important role because Generation Y does not see itself as 'order takers' or 'task executors' [emphasis in original]" (Werther, 2015, p. 8).

With the help of 360° feedback, not only can commitment and loyalty to the practice be promoted, but the diagnostic function can also be used to correctly assess the skills of employees so that they can be deployed appropriately . Practice managers can also analyse which skills are still lacking in the practice. The analysis can then lead to the practice management initiating further training measures tailored to the individual employees.

The core of this book is the creation of a feedback form for assessing the performance of therapists for patients and instructions for all those involved in the assessment. To this end, the second chapter of this book first examines the assessment of employees in general and in therapeutic practices in particular. It should be noted here that the underlying literature generally refers to commercial enterprises. The third chapter explains 360° feedback and the conditions for its introduction. The fourth chapter deals extensively with assessment by patients. The criteria and layout of the patient questionnaire are explained and justified. The questionnaire itself can be requested from the author if required. The fifth chapter deals with instructions for all those involved in the feedback process. Examples of instructions are provided here. The last and sixth chapter deals with the evaluation of the feedback.

CHAPTER 2

Employee assessment in therapeutic practices

According to Becker (2009, p. 165), the basic idea behind employee appraisals is to describe an observable actual performance result and compare it with a target result. This is not always about recording performance alone, but also about recording relevant personality traits and human impact (Jung 2011, p. 739). The latter is particularly important for therapeutic practices, as contact with patients is characterised by the human impact of the individual. Furthermore, work performance in therapeutic practices cannot be measured and quantified in the same way as in many other sectors of the economy. In addition, according to Sausele-Beyer (2011, p. 317), employees in social professions identify with both their field of expertise and their work with patients and therefore strive for further development themselves. In addition to operational and economic considerations, the purpose of employee assessment is also to provide individual advice, support and development for employees (Jung 2011, p. 739, 304). Schuler (1991, p. 14, cited in Nerdinger, 2014, p. 201) also formulates the goals of performance improvement and personnel development as well as personnel planning and personnel decisions, such as work assignments, promotions or dismissals, and even the design of working conditions. This last aspect can thus also lead to health prevention measures.

In order for performance appraisals to be carried out in the tightly scheduled workflow of therapeutic practices, they must be feasible in terms of time and personnel. Jung (2011, p. 782) sees the higher personnel requirements and greater time expenditure for supervisors as disadvantages of personnel appraisal. However, these are offset by the advantages of increased work productivity, potentially fairer remuneration, the possibility of acting in a more goal-oriented manner and the visibility of over- or under-challenging tasks for employees (ibid.).

A synonym for performance appraisal in the literature is performance review. Jung (2011, p. 304) distinguishes between economic and educational performance review. Jung (2011, p. 304) describes economic performance review as an "intangible investment in human capital". Current expenditure, e.g. arising from the time commitment of managers and employees, is incurred with the intention of generating future income (ibid.). This is the case when the special skills of employees are recorded so that they can be deployed in a targeted manner and the practice can offer an expanded range of services, for example. Educational performance monitoring includes personnel development, in which employees are given the opportunity to recognise their strengths and develop their skills and competencies (Jung, 2011, p. 305). Educational performance monitoring can take place by determining the degree of learning achievement with the help of self-monitoring and external monitoring as well as objective and subjective checks of the results (Jung 2011, p. 306). The possibility of self-assessment also means that educational performance monitoring meets the need for self-fulfilment expressed by Parment (2013, p. 157) for Generations Y and Z. However, the requirements for performance assessments vary depending on the objective of the assessment.

2.1 Requirements for performance assessments

Becker (2009, p. 284) formulates transparency, flexibility, comparability, cost-effectiveness and practicability as general requirements for performance appraisal procedures. A performance appraisal procedure is transparent if the participants are informed about the criteria, the process and the consequences in a timely manner. It is flexible if it takes into account the different tasks of the employees. An assessment procedure can be considered comparable if the same procedure is carried out in the same way for all employees. Assessment procedures can only be described as practical and economical if they can be carried out easily alongside other tasks within a reasonable time and with reasonable effort.

In order to assess an employee's actual performance appropriately, the procedure should relate to the specific tasks of the employee. Knowledge of the tasks and assessment criteria is important for the performance of the job. An assessment must also be situation- and time-related and be repeated. If tasks have changed during the reassessment, they must be re-described. Functional relevance requires that there must be different assessment tools for different tasks and functions. In order to do justice to employees with different qualifications, a performance appraisal must ultimately also be employee-related. This is particularly important for personnel development measures and educational personnel development (Becker, 2009, p. 282f).

The professional requirements of the employee are determined by observing and evaluating their performance. In doing so, the personality of the employee, as well as their talents and motivations, must be recognised and compared with the requirements of the job. Those conducting the assessment need to be good judges of character and should be as free as possible from prejudice, rigid thinking and dogmatism. The legal requirements for employee assessment are set out in the Works Constitution Act (Betriebsverfassungsgesetz) in Sections 81, which covers the obligation to provide information and discuss matters, the right to be heard and to discuss matters, the right to inspect personnel files ( ), the right to lodge complaints and the right of co-determination of the staff council (Jung 2011, p. 740f). The Lower Saxony Personnel Representation Act (NPersVG) also stipulates the co-determination of assessment criteria in Section 65 (1). According to Jung (2011, p. 742), employee assessments should be carried out at regular intervals in order to review the employee's development. It is recommended that they be repeated annually. In addition, an additional assessment may be carried out on special occasions, such as the end of the probationary period, an upcoming transfer or change in the employee's area of responsibility, or at the employee's request (ibid.).

However, if the assessment is a support measure, the focus should not be on measurable and comparable results (Becker, 2009, p. 278). Performance can then be considered in terms of different performance requirements, such as qualifications, abilities, skills, knowledge, motives and expectations. For example, an employee who has taught themselves new skills may have achieved more than an employee who has undergone further training in this area, even if the result of the good therapy is the same for both. Since the aim of performance assessment as a support measure is not to compare employees with each other, the different efforts made by employees to achieve the performance can be taken into account (Becker, 2009, p. 281f). This is also evident in the different types of assessment.

2.2 Types of assessment

Jung (2011, p. 738f) distinguishes between performance assessment and potential assessment. While performance assessment primarily serves management policy objectives, such as dismissals or promotions, the purpose of potential assessment is more related to personnel development, i.e. the further development of the employee. While performance assessment focuses on past performance, potential assessment is future-oriented and can result in a plan for further training or support measures (Jung, 2011, p. 738f).

Methodologically, a distinction is made between summary and analytical procedures. In summary procedures, performance is assessed as a whole. This includes free, open assessment that does not specify any categories or criteria for the assessment. Analytical procedures involve individual criteria that are combined to form an overall assessment (Jung, 2011, p. 753f). Analytical procedures thus enable a comparison of the assessment across different criteria. Jung (ibid.) also distinguishes between quantitative and qualitative procedures. In qualitative procedures, those providing feedback should describe the observed performance in their own words on the basis of questions, while quantitative procedures usually use a points system. The points system offers the possibility of a salary increase or other non-monetary benefits upon reaching a specified number of points (ibid.).

Becker (2009, p. 284ff) distinguishes between assessments using the ranking method, the labelling method, the classification method, task-oriented and goal-oriented assessment methods. In the ranking method, the feedback providers establish a ranking, i.e. a hierarchy between different feedback recipients. In labelling procedures, various possible behavioural options in a situation are described, which the feedback providers are asked to tick off, e.g. in a checklist procedure. In classification procedures, criteria are formulated, the achievement of which is documented on numerical or verbal scales. In task-oriented and goal-oriented assessment procedures ( ), a previously set task or goal is reviewed and evaluated. The latter is closely related to the concept *of management by objectives.* In this concept, which is very common in business, an economically oriented goal (e.g. 50 new customers) is formulated together with the employee. Achieving this goal is then rewarded, for example, with a salary increase, a promotion or a share in profits (ibid., p. 328).

Jung (2011, p. 754ff) formulates different levels of personnel assessment. For example, an employee can assess themselves and be assessed by superiors and peers (ibid.). Assessment by peers is particularly common in project groups. Here, employees are assessed by all members of the group (Nerdinger, 2014, p. 203f). As a rule, assessment by peers takes place in a standardised form (ibid., p. 205). When all these perspectives are taken into account at the same time and even customers and suppliers are involved, this is referred to as 360° feedback (Jung, 2011, p. 762ff). Jung (2011, p. 762) even presents an extension to 540° feedback, in which family members, life partners and friends can also provide feedback. The costs and effort involved in these different options vary greatly.

2.3 Benefits and effort involved in assessment

Employee appraisals serve the goals of the practice and those of the employees themselves. In addition to the desired increase in performance and thus turnover, operational goals include the objectification of human resources work. This allows the results of different employees to be compared, their potential assessed and utilised. Employees can assess their own work and thus plan their careers independently (Jung, 2011, p. 742f), e.g. by formulating wishes for further training. Practice managers can analyse the competence pool of their practice by assessing and promoting their employees and, if necessary, expand it in line with market requirements.

Employees can be encouraged to engage in self-reflection by comparing external assessments with their own self-image, thereby arriving at a more realistic self-assessment without "blind spots" (Scherm, Sarges, 2002, p. 3). This, in turn, can lead to further personal development. Dietzsch and Kaschube (2007, p. 16) also see the advantage for employees in receiving recognition for their work if the assessment is positive. Jung (2011, p. 743) notes that employees can use the subsequent discussion with their superiors to address their own concerns, e.g. training requests. In addition, appraisals offer a certain degree of protection against unjustified dismissals or arbitrary disciplinary measures, as employees can always refer to their most recent appraisal (ibid.).

In an evaluation meeting, the results of the assessment must be summarised and explained verbally if they are to have any effect. Employees should also have the opportunity to ask questions (Runde et al., 2001, p. 154f). According to Brenner (2015, p. 4), it is essential to set targets for the next assessment period.

A meta-analysis of 131 publications shows that performance improves with an effect size of d = .41 after feedback (Scherm, Sarges, 2002, p. 39). This means that the effect can be considered small to medium. Werther (2015, p. 15) emphasises that it is necessary to repeat feedback at intervals in order to improve performance. Furthermore, the results must not only be summarised in writing, but also communicated (ibid., p. 55).

The time required for employee assessment depends on the method chosen and the length of the questionnaire (Edwards, Ewen, 2000, p. 118f). For example, assessment by a superior or a peer alone is less time-consuming than assessment using 360° feedback. Formulating free text in a summary procedure is also more time-consuming than assessment using a criteria-based analytical procedure. The effort to avoid errors in the assessment is also a time factor.

2.4 Sources of error in assessment

The highest possible degree of objectivity can be achieved if sources of error are eliminated or at least minimised. Jung (2011, p. 765ff) distinguishes between perception errors, evaluation errors and consistency errors. Perception errors can occur even when observing performance, such as the exclusive perception of desired performance. Prejudices can also influence the perception of performance (ibid., p. 765f).

Similarly, the evaluation of performance is subject to various sources of error. For example, in *the halo effect*, performance can be overshadowed by other positive characteristics of the employee. The *one-sidedness effect* describes the assessment of overall performance, whether positive or negative, based on one outstanding event. In *transfer errors*, previous evaluations are adopted prematurely without critical examination. *The contact effect* refers to the fact that the more regular the contact between the evaluator and the employee, the better the employee's performance is assessed. The *Santa Claus effect* describes a better assessment due to special efforts made by the employee shortly before the assessment. The assessment error *Taking into account assessment consequences* leads to more positive assessments if the feedback recipient fears reprisals, such as salary cuts, as a result of the assessment. The *hierarchy effect* describes a better assessment of higher-ranking employees (ibid., p. 766f). In *the Andorra phenomenon*, the employee actually performs worse due to the negative opinion of their superior. The *stickiness effect* refers to a more negative assessment due to a lack of promotion in the past (ibid., p. 768f).

Errors that can be attributed to the personality structure of the evaluator are called consistency errors. This can result in evaluators who are too strict, too lenient, too cautious or too extreme (ibid., p. 768f). Finally, there is the tendency towards the middle, i.e. the tendency to give average ratings, and the tendency towards extreme ratings (ibid., p. 769f).

According to Becker (2009, p. 239), another bias to which assessors are subject is bias due to the therapist's self-presentation. Automatic processes include, for example, first impressions. Implicit personality assumptions are reflected, for example, in the type of clothing worn. A therapist who is dressed appropriately in the eyes of the assessor may therefore be considered more competent and subsequently receive a better assessment. This may lead to targeted, controlled behaviour on the part of the therapist in order to influence the assessment (ibid.). This bias is essentially another argument in favour of 360° feedback, as it brings together many different perspectives. For example, a therapist may receive a good rating from patients due to their friendly nature or appropriate clothing, but superiors and peers may see significant shortcomings in their professional competence. Therapists may even try to influence the assessors through controlled behaviour patterns. Discovering this requires a high degree of familiarity with assessment situations, which cannot be expected from patients and must be taken into account when assessing patients.

Becker (2009, p. 136) also explains a distortion of assessment results due to the assessment of memories stored in the memory. This occurs when the assessors do not assess the performance immediately after observation. When memorising the performance, it is not the behaviour that is evaluated, but the interpreted categorisation of the behaviour stored in memory (ibid.). This is a major difficulty with feedback forms for patients. They have experienced the therapists in several therapy situations and are asked to give a summary assessment at the end of the therapy. Patients therefore only evaluate their subjective and interpreted memory of the performance. If the feedback form is distributed at the beginning of therapy and the criteria are already known, this distortion cannot be prevented, but it can at least be reduced, as patients may be able to assign behaviour more quickly to the criteria they are already familiar with and, if necessary, store the performance in the categories used in the feedback form. This bias must also be taken into account in feedback forms for supervisors and peers. However, the longer the procedure is used, the more familiar the feedback providers are with the criteria, so that this bias becomes less significant.

All feedback providers are subject to the assessment errors mentioned above. While therapists and supervisors have more knowledge about possible assessment errors due to their training, most patients will not have had any experience with them. However, knowledge about possible assessment errors reduces the likelihood of them occurring. Unfortunately, this methodological weakness of feedback cannot be remedied.

CHAPTER 3

360° feedback and its relevance for the therapeutic professions

360° feedback, also known as all-round assessment, is a "systematic, formalised and largely standardised descriptive or evaluative assessment of employees in a company (feedback recipients)" (Jung, 2011, p. 762). In the United States, 360° feedback is also known as multisource feedback or multi-rater feedback (Scherm, Sarges, 2002, p. 3). The purpose of 360° feedback is to gather employee-related performance information from different perspectives, i.e. from different people. Like any assessment tool, it can be used to improve employee motivation and skills in terms of personnel development, as well as for management and personnel policy purposes (Jung, 2011, p. 762f). According to Scherm and Sarges (2002, p. 3), 360° feedback is one of the psychologically based personnel assessment and personnel development tools. In business, 360° feedback is increasingly used in the USA and in larger companies (Scherm, Sarges, 2002, p. 7). American Airlines, for example, has been using 360° feedback since 1987 (Edwards, Ewen, 2000, p. 129).
According to Werther (2015, p. 46), 360° feedback should be introduced by experts. Unlike in large companies, this is not absolutely necessary in therapeutic practices due to their small, more manageable size. It also involves costs and is therefore unlikely to be practised by practices.

360° feedback is carried out in four phases. In the first phase, the goals of the feedback are defined, the boundary conditions are checked and the instrument is selected. In the second phase, employees are informed in a transparent manner and the data is collected. The third phase involves evaluating the results and providing feedback to the feedback recipients. The fourth and final phase involves initiating follow-up measures, such as further training (Scherm,

Sarges, 2002, p. 47ff).

The four phases of 360° feedback have already been partially achieved through the theoretical work presented here. The first phase includes setting goals, reviewing conditions and selecting the instrument. The goals of feedback, namely personnel development and planning further measures, have already been described in this book. The instruments, in particular the feedback form for patients, have been selected or designed. The form already in use in practice can be used as an assessment form for self-assessment and assessment by superiors and peers. Additional forms can be purchased in the supplementary material to the book "Praxis-Management für Physiotherapeuten, Ergotherapeuten und Logopäden" (Practice Management for Physiotherapists, Occupational Therapists and Speech Therapists) by Barbara Betz. During this phase, the practice should check the conditions: Who will participate in the feedback? How will the data be collected (online or on paper)? How and by whom will the feedback be evaluated? How will the anonymity of the participants be ensured? In what time frame should the feedback take place (total duration)? How often should it be repeated?

The second phase involves informing employees and collecting data. If practices do not want to or cannot use service providers to evaluate the results, the third phase will be very time-consuming for the practices. If Excel spreadsheets are used for evaluation, those evaluating the data should have a certain level of understanding of the programme. Sufficient time must also be allocated. It is certainly critical to consider whether supervisors should carry out the evaluation themselves. In a small team in particular, it can happen that " " assessments are attributed to peers. If the practice has a service employee in the reception area, they could take over the evaluation, i.e. entering the results into an existing Excel spreadsheet. In this case, supervisors only receive the summary, and the assignment of assessments to employees can be minimised. The fourth phase involves initiating goals and measures and must be carried out by supervisors or practice management in consultation with employees.

3.1 The levels of 360° feedback

The focus of the feedback is on the feedback recipients. The vertical level refers to feedback from supervisors and subordinate employees (Werther, 2015, p. 22). Originally, 360° feedback was used to evaluate supervisors in larger companies (Scherm, Sarges, 2002, p. 4). However, as the management levels in therapeutic practices tend to be flat, it is usually not possible for employees to receive feedback from subordinates, unless the feedback recipients are the practice managers. They could also receive feedback on their leadership qualities (Edwards, Ewen, 2000, p. 56).

The horizontal level of 360° feedback includes assessment by peers and patients as external customers (Werther, 2015, p. 22f). The role of patients has changed significantly in recent decades. The empowerment movement, which encourages people to make more self-determined health decisions, is leading to a decline in the dominance of healthcare professions (Naidoo, Wills, 2003, p. 80). In their role as customers, patients demand a say and information (Schmacke, 2005, p. 167). They decide on the therapy and the practice within certain parameters specified by the health insurance companies. Against this background, it is only logical to allow them to participate in the evaluation of their therapist.

Those receiving feedback also assess their own performance and can then compare their self-assessment with the different assessments at the various levels. To this end, it is important that the same instruments are used wherever possible (Nerdinger, 2014, p. 207). Here, it is possible for feedback recipients to complete both the subject-specific feedback form for supervisors and peers and the feedback form for patients for their self-assessment.

If the assessments of superiors and peers differ greatly, Becker (2009, p. 230f) recommends controlled observation. This would mean that specific situations in therapy are observed by both superiors and peers. However, this is an unnatural situation that is similar to an examination. The extent to which therapists would then display behaviour typical of them is questionable. The St. Nicholas effect (see section 2.4) may occur. Nevertheless, a solution must be found in the event of recurring, contradictory or strongly divergent assessments. A team meeting with all those involved would also be possible, although anonymity would not be maintained in this case.

3.2 Use for personnel policy purposes or as personnel development?

According to Becker (2009, p. 380), assessment tools should not be used simultaneously for advisory purposes, i.e. for personnel development, and for personnel policy purposes, e.g. as a basis for salary increases. Supervisors would find themselves in role conflicts, as they would have to take on both the role of coach and that of judge (Edwards, Ewen, 2000, p. 22). Edwards and Ewen (, 2000, p. 67f) are critical of the use of 360° feedback in performance appraisal for personnel policy purposes. They argue that evaluations by peers tend to be too positive, as employees do not want to harm their colleagues or hinder their careers (ibid.). It is also possible to manipulate the system, for example through collusion. These problems can be countered by removing absolute anonymity, e.g. by using an identification number on the feedback form, which enables the evaluators to trace forms that have been filled in manipulatively (ibid., p. 68f).

Nerdinger (2014, p. 209) also states that 360° feedback should only be used for personal development. If 360° feedback is nevertheless used in performance appraisal for personnel policy purposes, it is subject to higher requirements. The link to the work must be clearly established, the criteria must be valid, legal issues must be taken into account, and sources of error must be analysed and eliminated (Edwards, Ewen, 2000, p. 64). There are also a number of arguments in favour of using it in performance assessment for personnel policy purposes. For example, 360° feedback is fair, accurate and useful for personal development (Edwards, Ewen, 2000, p. 29), and its effectiveness has been proven in many studies (Dietzsch-Kley, Ka- schube, 2007, p. 4). The multi-perspective feedback provides employees with a holistic assessment of their skills and performance in all situations and tasks that are important for their job (Edwards, Ewen, 2000, p. 20). This complements the assessment by the supervisor and, where necessary, puts problems with supervisor assessment, such as personal bias, favouritism, lack of observation opportunities and differing interpretations of the situations observed, into perspective, thereby preventing a possible career setback due to misjudgement (Edwards, Ewen, 2000, p. 19). Misjudgements can result in the wrong people being appointed to positions and tasks, economic failure, tensions within the team and a loss of motivation among employees (Jung, 2011, p. 771 f). In a generation in which work is increasingly seen as less of a duty and loyalty to employers is declining, loss of motivation is a particular reason for changing jobs (Parment 2013, p. 58f). However, this is precisely what must be prevented in therapeutic practices, as the shortage of skilled workers is already very noticeable here.

Employees are often better able to accept feedback from several different assessors, as the credibility of the statements increases due to the multi-perspective view. It is irrelevant whether the assessment is carried out for personnel policy purposes or for personnel development. In addition, colleagues are more likely to address poor performance with employees than supervisors are (Edwards, Ewen, 2000, p. 30f). Furthermore, "colleagues (...) can assess the contributions of each individual employee much more competently (...)" (Nerdinger, 2014, p. 204). p. 30f). Furthermore, "colleagues (...) are much better able to assess the contributions of each individual employee (...)" (Nerdinger, 2014, p. 204). Jung (2011, p. 759f) emphasises that peers can only assess an employee's performance if they are informed about the employee's tasks and goals and have had sufficient opportunity to observe their behaviour. The assessors must also have the necessary professional competence (ibid.).

In therapeutic practices, performance appraisals for personnel policy purposes are generally less common, partly because career opportunities tend to be limited. In addition, as a social enterprise, a practice tends to have a family-like structure (Sausele-Beyer, 2011, p. 144). Supervisors in social enterprises therefore tend to support their employees more than they control them (Sausele-Beyer, 2011, p. 98). The advantages of 360° feedback for therapeutic practices therefore lie more in personnel development.

3.3 Advantages

In addition to personnel development, the advantages of 360° feedback for therapeutic practices lie primarily in customer loyalty. Patients feel that they are taken seriously and are given a voice. They are thus indirectly involved in decisions and directly involved in quality control. They also have the opportunity to contribute their own ideas for improvement (Edwards, Ewen, 2000, p. 21ff).

The task of practice management is to ensure economic success, including by ensuring the quality of therapy (Betz, 2014, p. 2). According to Jung (2011, p. 306), one way of monitoring success and thus ensuring quality is to evaluate employees. Superiors receive valuable information via 360° feedback to help them fulfil their management tasks (Edwards, Ewen, 2000, p. 21ff) and thus maintain their practice's position in the market. According to Edwards and Ewen (2000, p. 24f), another advantage is that many assessments are obtained from different perspectives. Practice managers themselves often have only limited opportunities to observe the performance of their employees, as they are usually not present during therapy.

The 360° feedback with its multi-perspective view can also be used to determine whether further training measures are having an effect on patients (Scherm, Sarges, 2002, p. 7). Scherm and Sarges (2002, p. 9) describe 360° feedback as a change "on the job" that can bridge the transfer gap, as the feedback is based on a specific professional situation. The transfer gap refers to the problem of not using a qualification obtained through further education or training, for example (Jung, 2011, p. 308f).

For employees, the advantages of 360° feedback include increased motivation, as performance can be rewarded through participation in further development (Edwards, Ewen, 2000, p. 21 f). For example, training courses can be tailored more precisely to the development needs and wishes of individuals, and ideas for change can be introduced (, Scherm, Sarges, 2002, p. 9).

Parment (2013, p. 157) also addresses the socio-cultural side of the social changes already mentioned. According to him, Generations Y and Z are characterised by certain expectations: while earlier generations saw their job primarily as a means of securing their livelihood, the needs of the current generation tend to lie in self-fulfilment and co-determination. Since 360° feedback via surveys and evaluations offers the opportunity for participation and co-determination in important decisions within the company (Gerpott, 2013, p. 134), it is also an argument for attracting potential employees, according to Werther (2015, p. 35). Employees can evaluate their peers as team members and also receive feedback on their own behaviour and skills (Edwards, Ewen, 2000, p. 21ff). Sausele-Beyer (2011, p. 318) also notes that employees in social enterprises strive for development because they generally identify strongly with the company and its social activities. "The close link between the individual and their professional competence also results in a commitment and actual responsibility for their own personal and professional development" (ibid., p. 318). Scherm and Sarges (2002, p. 14) also see feedback as a driver for change and self-fulfilment, as we learn from experience. "It is precisely the *reflection* on experiences and the evaluation of feedback that enables deeper learning processes – experience *alone [*emphasis in original] is not enough" (Tjosvold, 1991, no page number, quoted from Scherm and Sarges, 2002, p. 14).

The biggest disadvantage of 360° feedback, apart from the aforementioned possibilities of manipulation, is the time and cost factor. While assessment by superiors only ties up their own working time, 360° feedback involves all employees in the assessment process and means that those receiving feedback cannot treat patients during this time. The duration of the feedback varies depending on the length and complexity of the questionnaire. The larger the practice, the more employees have to be assessed, and the longer each individual employee needs for this. In addition, employees may find the additional task stressful. This is particularly true when it is used during periods of major change (Scherm, Sarges, 2002, p. 71). Scherm and Sarges (2002, p. 70) are of the opinion that the considerable effort involved in 360° feedback only makes sense if it has consequences for the employee, e.g. in the form of remuneration or non-monetary rewards. Further training, consideration of the employee's special wishes or other support from the practice owner can also fulfil this function. In any case, the objectives should be formulated jointly at the end and their achievement reviewed by the next feedback session. If 360° feedback is used during periods of major change, e.g. to enable better deployment of employees or to cut jobs for economic reasons, those giving feedback tend to be lenient because they do not want to harm their colleagues. Rater training, i.e. training employees in 360° feedback, is particularly important here (Scherm, Sarges, 2002, p. 71f). However, this incurs additional costs and is certainly difficult for practice owners to implement in times of tight budgets.Evaluating the results of 360° feedback is also more challenging and time-consuming due to the different levels and the need to highlight differences and similarities in the assessments if the findings are to be valid. Companies now offer online evaluation services. This topic will be discussed in more detail in Chapter Five.

3.4 Comparison with assessment by superiors

Compared to traditional assessments by supervisors, 360° feedback increases the accuracy of evaluations and supports a participatory corporate culture, teamwork and employee empowerment. (Edwards, Ewen, 2000, p. 75). While individual assessments by supervisors cement their absolute power, 360° feedback provides joint input. Blind evaluations and subjective assessments based on the assumption that supervisors possess assessment skills per se (Edwards, Ewen, 2000, p. 75) stand in the way of what Scherm and Sarges (2002, p. 1) call a "multi-perspective approach". However, it is wrong to assume that the assessment will be completely objective just because there are many evaluators (Nerdinger, 2014, p. 209). Becker (2009, p. 215) refers to this as intersubjectivity, which is close to objectivity. This is the degree of agreement between different subjective judgements. Depending on how many assessors there are and how much agreement there is, intersubjectivity always exists to varying degrees (ibid.). Several studies have shown that there is no sufficient correlation between self-assessment and peer assessment, or between self-assessment and supervisor assessment alone. An assessment that takes all perspectives into account equally therefore actually offers the person being assessed the opportunity to obtain additional information about their own performance and abilities (Gerpott, 2013, p. 135). This can be achieved using different methods of conducting 360° feedback.

3.5 Methods

Until now, written 360° feedback in the form of a feedback form has been assumed. However, 360° feedback, at least from the perspective of superiors and peers, can also be provided verbally, e.g. in team meetings. However, this carries the risk that team members will not be honest because they fear reprisals after the meeting. However, open feedback can also be helpful for team building ( ). Nevertheless, even with the anonymous written version, honest answers cannot be expected if employees feel that the information will not be treated confidentially (Edwards, Ewen, 2000, p. 48).

There are many options for presenting the questionnaires. In addition to the usual paper versions, password-protected online access (Dietzsch, Kaschube, 2007, p. 10) or software on company laptops or tablets (Edwards, Ewen, 2000, p. 228) can also be used. Password-protected online access has the advantage that patients can complete the evaluation at home at their leisure. However, this means that they may forget to fill it in.

Filling out feedback forms on a tablet or laptop offers the opportunity to make good use of waiting time at the practice, which also has the added benefit of ensuring a higher response rate for the feedback forms. However, participants may not be sure whether their evaluation will remain anonymous. In this case, the assessment may not be honest (Dietzsch, Kaschube, 2007, p. 8). To maintain anonymity, a special programme would have to be used that stores the contents of the completed form and immediately deletes it for the next assessment. To comply with data protection regulations, no other programmes or data should be present on the data carrier. This method of completion, together with password-protected online services, minimises costs, even if a one-off investment in software and laptops or tablets is required. Compared to questionnaires, this saves money on paper, printer ink and, if applicable, postage (Edwards and Ewen, 2000, p. 228). It should also be noted that this method prevents errors in the transfer of data for evaluation, as would be the case with paper versions. However, both digital variants require a certain level of technical media literacy on the part of those providing feedback. This cannot be assumed for all citizens.

Edwards and Ewen (2000) identify informal and formal systems for written feedback (p. 32f). While informal systems are quickly developed, individual systems of questioning or assessment, formal systems offer procedural guidelines that ensure fairness, anonymity and standardised evaluation methods. They are more time-consuming to develop and implement. Formal systems are also more expensive due to the need for technical equipment and training. Since informal systems do not include safeguards to guarantee a fair process, they should be rejected, especially when used for performance assessment (Edwards, Ewen, 2000, p. 32f). The following chapter presents the procedure for formal systems.

3.6 Procedure for introducing a formal system

According to Gerpott (2013, p. 132), 360° feedback fulfils two primary functions: diagnosis and behaviour modification. The diagnostic function is intended to enable employees to review their self-reflection by presenting their own strengths and weaknesses from different perspectives. These then enable the second primary function of behaviour modification. Based on the 360° feedback, employees can change their behaviour and performance in line with their own goals and those of the company (ibid.).

If you want to introduce 360° feedback, it is important to consider important details in advance. According to Edwards and Ewen (2000, p. 34), the process should be designed by the users. For example, assessment criteria for the feedback form must be identified and formulated by analysing the workplace and the tasks. "Only a *context-, goal- and assessor-oriented specification (...)* can *capture* the object (*or "the" performance)* in a way that is " " [emphasis in original] (Becker, 2009, p. 168).

In the case of feedback forms for self-assessment, assessment by superiors and peers, it would certainly be desirable for practices to involve employees as much as possible in the feedback process. For example, the team could decide whether the observation situations on which the feedback is based should be random or planned. This is particularly important because the extent to which colleagues are aware of each other's work is likely to vary from practice to practice. However, it should be noted that this also applies to supervisors. In most cases, they are not only supervisors but also colleagues, as they are usually involved in patient care in the practice.

In addition, the team could decide whether all patient feedback forms should be taken into account or whether a selection should be made, e.g. by month or at random. This will certainly also depend on the number of feedback forms received.

For valid 360° feedback, at least four additional assessors are required in addition to the supervisors and the employees themselves (Edwards, Ewen, 2000, p. 34). This is certainly not always the case in small practices. Whether 360° feedback can still be useful here depends on the attitude of the employees. If they see the feedback as an opportunity for change and a chance to pursue their own goals, the lack of validity can be accepted. However, this can also lead to a decrease in the anonymity of the feedback, which, according to Bortz et al. (2006, p. 257), can in turn lead to dishonest answers.

In order to compare the results of self-assessment, peer feedback and feedback from superiors, the same assessment form should be used (Nerdinger, 2014, p. 209). If there is already a form for assessing employees in practice with , this can be used for assessment by the practice management, peers and for self-assessment.

According to Edwards et al. (2000, p. 34), scientific and methodological criteria relating to surveys should be taken into account during data collection and evaluation. In the case of the feedback questionnaire for patients presented here, this can be assumed to be the case, as it was developed on the basis of an extensive survey of patients by Dehn-Hindenberg (2008) (see section 4.5). It should be noted critically that the survey was conducted in 2005 and the results could therefore be considered outdated. Unfortunately, I was unable to find any more recent surveys on this topic. However, I also believe that the needs of patients have not changed significantly over the last 10 years. Only the need for information may have decreased due to the wealth of information now available on the Internet. Nowadays, there may be a greater need to resolve uncertainties arising from information found on the Internet.

According to Edwards et al. (2000, p. 34), employees must also be trained in giving feedback and in the assessment process before 360° feedback is introduced. A short in-house refresher course would probably suffice here, as therapists have already learned how to give and receive feedback during their basic training.

After a trial run, the feedback process should be reviewed by users for fairness, transparency and accuracy (Edwards, Ewen, 2000, p. 34). This evaluation, which can also take place on an ongoing basis, is certainly possible in " " practices in the case of feedback from peers and superiors. The extent to which continuous evaluation of the feedback form by patients is possible is questionable, partly because patients change constantly and have not been involved in previous changes. This means that processes that have already been rejected in previous reviews may be resubmitted as suggestions.

Although the assessments should be requirement- and task-related and not focus on the personality of the employee, voluntary participation is part of the concept of 360° feedback. Employees should also be allowed to choose the people who give them feedback (Gerpott, 2013, p. 142f). According to Nerdinger (2014, p. 210f)[1] , employees also select critical individuals. Edwards and Ewen (2000, p. 213) even state that when there are friendly relationships between feedback providers and recipients, the assessment is often even more severe. With regard to feedback from peers, the selection of feedback providers should be viewed critically. Practices are usually not large enough to

[1] Note: Nerdinger quotes Gerpott (2006) here without specifying the page number. However, the passage marked here could only be found in part in the original literature cited or in the newer editions of the chapter of the same name from 2013, which are also cited here.

allow for selection. The voluntary nature of participation should also be viewed critically. What should a practice manager do

if employees refuse to participate, but the important data cannot be dispensed with? To what extent will forced feedback bring about the desired motivational boost and insights? A discussion within the team with a clear idea of the procedure and the advantages of feedback is certainly helpful here. However, the use of 360° feedback is questionable if there is resistance from employees.

During the implementation and evaluation, absolute anonymity must be ensured. The evaluation should be carried out by experts. It is important to create a summary of the assessment from the various perspectives. The summary is handed to the employee. Under no circumstances should it be filed in the personnel file (Nerdinger, 2014, p. 210f)[1].

In order to prevent dissatisfaction with the 360° feedback process, the evaluation of the feedback must be followed by a discussion and, ideally, measures and goals should be set and initiated (Edwards, Ewen, 2000, p. 186).

CHAPTER 4

Evaluation by patients

4.1 Patients as customers

In recent decades, the role of patients has increasingly changed from that of ignorant people in need of help to partners with a say in the treatment process. This was already described in 1986 by the WHO's Ottawa Charter. According to this, people should be empowered to take a greater degree of self-determination in their own healing process (Ottawa Charter 1986). This process is also known as empowerment. In occupational therapy, the client-centred approach, which also promotes participation, is considered the paradigm for treatment. In Germany, this approach was further consolidated by the legislation of SGB IX and the introduction of the participation-oriented ICF (Flotho, 2015, p. 200f). Patient participation is therefore expressly desired; they should be seen as customers or clients. However, Dehn-Hindenberg (2008, p. 111) notes that many other characteristics of customers are not present. For example, patients do not have a free choice of healthcare services, as these are based on the diagnosed illness and the health insurance companies' offer to cover the costs. Customer rights, such as the right to exchange goods if they are not satisfactory, are also not guaranteed (ibid.). Patients are therefore not customers in the true sense of the market economy. Nevertheless, they are co-decision-makers and are increasingly demanding this in medicine (Schmacke, 2005, p. 167).

According to Betz (2014, p. 53), the needs-based and economical care of patients and the transparency of treatment outcomes are essential factors in quality management in healthcare. While quality management systems must already be proven for certification in the inpatient sector, this is currently only mandatory in the outpatient sector for service providers who provide preventive care in a health resort (ibid.). According to Bruhn (2013, p. 115), the main task of quality management in the service sector is to tailor company performance to customer requirements. Service quality can therefore be measured using customer-oriented measurement approaches, which include customer surveys (ibid.). Customer-oriented measurement approaches can be divided into differentiated and undifferentiated approaches. Undifferentiated measurement approaches only obtain global satisfaction ratings. Only differentiated measurement approaches allow detailed statements to be made about partial qualities (Bruhn, 2013, p. 117). The patient questionnaire developed to evaluate therapists is one of the differentiated, subjective and feature-oriented approaches, as it assesses individual customers' views of the therapists' performance using features that are relevant to the patients (Bruhn, 2013, p. 123).

Following the line of thinking of customer orientation and customer participation, it is entirely legitimate to give patients a say in the assessment of their therapist. However, due to the fact that, despite all the knowledge they may have acquired about their illness, they are not experts in the medical sense, the assessment criteria must be linked to the therapist's abilities that can be assessed by them. This may be the reason why existing instruments for patient feedback often do not include an assessment of the therapist.

4.2 Existing instruments

As already mentioned, many practices use patient questionnaires. The forms are usually designed by the practices themselves and have never been evaluated, so they cannot be considered standardised. Some practices use the feedback form from the Institute for Quality Assurance for Healthcare Providers (IQH). Although this form partly addresses the communication skills of the therapists, it cannot be traced back to the therapist if the form is filled out anonymously, as the name of the therapist is not mentioned. As a rule, the forms ask about the quality of the structure as well as the quality of the process and results. Freely written comments are often allowed.The feedback form for patients developed in this book, on the other hand, allows not only the communication and therapeutic relationship to be assessed, but also many other items. This enables the patient to evaluate the planning and organisation of the therapy by the therapist, the guidance and the therapy itself, as well as the outcome. In addition to structural quality, the process and outcome quality of the therapy are also assessed.

4.3 Structural quality, process quality and outcome quality

In order to assess the quality of a service, it can be evaluated according to its structural quality, process quality and outcome quality. Objective structural quality refers, for example, to personnel and practical resources, while personal structural quality refers to the professional and psychosocial methodological competence of employees (Betz, 2014, p. 54; Dehn-Hindenberg, 2008, p. 72). Personal structural quality is important for patients to assess the performance of employees. Patients are usually unable to assess professional competence, although according to Barth (1999, p. 483ff), it should contribute to building trust between the therapist and the patient. Psychosocial methodological competence, on the other hand, determines the diversity of interpersonal behaviour in the therapeutic relationship and is therefore particularly important in difficult situations. Process quality includes, for example, the procedures in the practice and the quality of treatment, including the actual communicative and psychosocial behaviour of the therapist. The latter contribute significantly to patient satisfaction and thus to customer loyalty (Dehn-Hindenberg, 2008, p. 73). The quality of results also looks at patient satisfaction and treatment success (Betz, 2014, p. 54). The quality of results can provide clear indications of necessary quality assurance measures in a therapeutic practice. Satisfied customers not only return, but also act as multipliers, for example when asked by acquaintances about a good practice (Philipsen, 2007, p. 3; Dehn-Hindenberg, 2008, p. 73). This patient-oriented view of quality is only indirectly reflected in this three-part structure of process, structure and outcome quality. Barth (1999, p. 328) adds this as a fourth, independent dimension.

4.4 Questionnaire development

Developing a questionnaire is a lengthy and difficult process if you want to achieve validity in terms of content (Edwards, Ewen, 2000, p. 100). An impression of the complexity can be gained by looking at the conditions to which, for example, the criteria of a questionnaire are subject. Criteria should be able to describe the object of the performance accurately and precisely (Becker, 2009, p. 167). They are subject to various quality criteria (Becker, 2009, p. 170). Content validity is given if the underlying observation can be considered representative of the performance behaviour shown (Becker, 2009, p. 172). Content validity, if at all, can only be assessed by experts in a logical analysis (Becker, 2009, p. 177f). The criteria of the feedback form for patients were largely developed from a survey of over 600 patients with functional disorders ( ) conducted by Dehn-Hindenberg (2008) in therapeutic practices. Patients can be regarded as experts in their own needs. Due to the large number of patients surveyed, the results can be considered relevant and the criteria valid and reliable. Nevertheless, the criteria of the feedback questionnaire should be pre-tested in therapeutic practices. According to Becker (2009, p. 177f), constant review of the criteria, the questionnaire and the process is necessary, but empirical testing to increase validity is hardly possible in practice (Becker, 2009, p. 177f). This applies in particular to therapeutic practices, which, unlike large commercial companies, do not have the necessary resources to do so.

Intra-individual judgement concordance or self-concordance refers to a high degree of agreement between observations made at different points in time (Becker, 2009, p. 170). Inter-individual judgement consistency is particularly important during 360° feedback. It means that different assessors should evaluate the criterion in the same way (Becker, 2009, p. 170f). "However, complete agreement between the assessments of the assessors cannot be expected" (Becker, 2009, p. 176). The reason for this lies in the lack of self-concordance. An assessment of the same behaviour by the same feedback provider can lead to different assessments at different times (ibid.). According to Edwards and Ewen (2000, p. 157), 360° feedback is meaningful if less than 5% of the feedback providers deviate by more than 20% from the consensus of the assessment group. In addition, 70% of the feedback providers should have given nearly identical assessments (ibid.). It can be assumed that a wide range of assessments is an indication that employees are perceived very differently, have behaved inconsistently towards different feedback providers, or that the tasks or observable situations are not very comparable. Individual outliers in the assessment are possible, however, also due to errors in judgement.

Finally, according to Becker (2009, p. 174), the relevance of the criterion for the work area must be considered. Individual criteria can be linked to work performance, but often not directly to the success of the company (ibid.). In therapeutic practices, for example, success could be measured in relation to the number of patients who not only choose the same practice for a second treatment, but even request the same employee.

The criteria in the questionnaire should be short, clear and actively formulated. The statements represent the competencies and should be formulated as unambiguously as possible. Individual competencies can be specified in more detail by second-degree competencies (Edwards, Ewen, 2000, p. 100f); Becker (2009, p. 189f) refers to these as subcriteria. Subcriteria describe an important aspect of the competence being assessed. According to Becker (2009, p. 347f), everyone defines the meaning of criteria slightly differently. They are therefore ambiguous, imprecise and flexible. For maximum validity, the questionnaire should therefore be checked by users in a preliminary test for readability, completeness and comprehensibility. The users' experiences should then be continuously incorporated so that the questionnaire and the process can be evaluated on an ongoing basis (Edwards Ewen, 2000, p. 106).

The criteria in the questionnaire should also be reliable. Reliability is achieved when the questions or criteria are understood in the same way by different people under different survey conditions (Porst, 2014, p. 17).

The scale should be fairly wide. Edwards and Ewen (2000, p. 116ff) recommend a 10-point scale. Narrower scales result in a flat profile, while broader scales allow strengths and weaknesses to be identified more clearly ( ). Both evaluators and those being evaluated prefer broader scales, as this increases motivation to change behaviour (ibid.). Scales anchored with descriptive sentences help to understand the scale (Edwards, Ewen, 2000, p. 111). However, caution is advised here with non-native speakers. Understanding of the criteria may be limited. Even translated forms do not always accurately reflect the content of the criteria. In addition, what is considered an acceptable rating varies from culture to culture (Edwards, Ewen, 2000, p. 113). "While it is perfectly acceptable to receive an average rating in one country, in another country it is unthinkable and is immediately understood by employees as a request to resign" (Dietzsch-Kley, Kaschube, 2007, p. 10). Furthermore, it cannot be guaranteed that all people from other cultural backgrounds, regardless of the length of their stay in our country, understand the German language well enough to grasp the meaning of the criteria. The same applies to a lesser extent to educational differences within the native German-speaking population. This must be taken into account when evaluating the feedback.

The questionnaire should not be too long. Patients are more willing to complete a questionnaire if the time required to do so is reasonable. It is therefore important to indicate in advance how long it is likely to take to complete the questionnaire (Bortz, Döring, 2006, p. 257). In the case of colleagues, the length of the questionnaire is also relevant because they usually have to complete several questionnaires. There should be no more than 35 criteria on the questionnaire. On average, respondents answer 3 questions in one minute. After 15 minutes, fatigue sets in, which may lead to misjudgement or non-evaluation of the criterion (Edwards, Ewen, 2000, p. 118f).

4.5 Criteria of the feedback form for patients according to Dehn-Hindenberg

Despite all the knowledge they may have acquired about their illness, patients are not experts in the medical sense. An assessment of the therapist's performance must therefore be linked to the therapist's assessable skills.

According to Becker (2009, p. 184f), criteria should not be selected solely on the basis of availability, e.g. existing questionnaires, but after careful analysis of the tasks and the workplace. Dehn-Hindenberg (2008) evaluated 665 questionnaires from patients of therapeutic practices in the fields of occupational therapy, physiotherapy and speech therapy. Due to the size of the sample and the analysis of the data in terms of reliability, validity, factor analysis and Bonferroni error calculation, the data obtained can be considered meaningful. The survey focuses on patients' needs in terms of communication and interaction, e.g. explanations and instructions, and their assessment of the therapy content. Key factors in interaction were individual information, determining the course of therapy, and empathetic, communicative and humorous behaviour (Dehn-Hindenberg, 2008, p. 164f).

No questions were asked about the factual structural quality, i.e. general services such as the provision of parking spaces.

The focus was on the personal structural quality of the therapists, i.e. their interpersonal skills with patients and the patients' satisfaction with these (Dehn-Hindenberg, 2008, p. 158).

When needs and wishes are satisfied, satisfaction arises. In the German encyclopaedia " Lexikon Wahrig", *satisfied* is defined as "satisfied, (...) having no major wishes" (Wahrig, 1994, p. 1800). Patient satisfaction therefore means that the needs and wishes of patients are met and that they are satisfied with the treatment. This is a subjective feeling and varies from person to person. According to Dehn-Hindenberg (2008, p. 136), there does not have to be a direct connection between objective treatment modalities, such as the duration of treatment and technical equipment, and the individual assessment of these, as the factors that influence patient satisfaction are diverse (ibid.). The study by Beattie et al. on patient satisfaction in physiotherapy practices (2002, p. 563) found that patient satisfaction also depends on the quality of the therapeutic relationship and interactions. The duration of therapy, communication skills and empathetic listening are particularly noteworthy here (ibid.). Philipsen (2007, p. 99f) also identifies the therapeutic relationship as a key factor in patient satisfaction with medical care. In a survey of 206 adult patients, the most important factors were the time the doctor took for the patients, the information and explanations provided, and the responsiveness to the patient's personal situation (ibid.). However, the success of the treatment also contributes to satisfaction. A subjectively or objectively improved state of health leads to more satisfied patients (Philipsen, 2007, p. 10).
However, in order to meet patient needs, these must be known in advance in the specific treatment context (Dehn-Hindenberg, 2008, p. 137). The treatment context in a hospital is generally different from that in a therapeutic practice, simply due to the severity of the illness. Furthermore, patient surveys from the medical field cannot be easily compared with those from a therapeutic practice. The context of the treatment is therefore important for the selection of evaluation criteria for assessing the performance of an employee. Dehn-

Hindenberg took precisely this into account in her survey of 665 patients from occupational therapy, physiotherapy and speech therapy practices.
Patients can evaluate the quality of communication, treatment processes, trust and the successful establishment of a therapeutic relationship. These criteria contribute significantly to recovery (Dehn-Hindenberg, 2008, p. 142). Communication, including the provision of information to patients, is particularly important in this context. "The quality (...) and comprehensibility of information are particularly important determinants of a good therapy evaluation" (Dehn-Hindenberg, 2008, p. 150).

For the present development of patient questionnaires as part of the 360° feedback from employees of therapeutic practices, the criteria that were most important for patients, i.e. those with the highest ratings, were selected from the Dehn-Hindenberg survey (Dehn-Hindenberg, 2008, p. 178ff). In the patient survey, Dehn-Hindenberg used a five-point Likert scale with a verbalised scale with endpoints. The highest rating was "*very important* (1)", the lowest "*not important*".

The statements in the patient feedback should refer to the highest ratings (1 = "= " and 2 = "*important*") in the survey. The most important criteria are listed below. The criteria are used to generate statements that patients can use to evaluate their therapists. The number of the statement in the feedback form is shown in brackets after each criterion (see section 4.7). Only criteria that were rated as very important or important by at least 75% of respondents were taken into account. This is an arbitrary value, but it represents the vast majority of respondents. In the feedback form developed for patients to evaluate their therapists, the statements are grouped into the following categories: planning and organisation of therapy, communication and therapeutic relationship, guidance and therapy, and outcome of therapy. According to Porst (2014, p. 99f), the statements should be formulated using simple, unambiguous terms so that all respondents understand them in the same way. The statements should not be too long or complex. Technical terms or foreign words should be avoided, and unclear terms should be explained if necessary (ibid.).

The results of the survey conducted by Dehn-Hindenberg are presented on the following pages. The feedback form created for patients, whose statements are listed in the next chapter, refers to this survey.

4.5.1 Therapy planning/participation

The patients surveyed considered joint therapy planning (see statement no. 1) to be very important or important, but still wanted the therapist to choose the therapy methods. A large number of patients, on the other hand, wanted the therapists to determine the therapy plan (Dehn-Hindenberg, 2008, p. 178f). Therapists can ask about this in the preliminary discussion or it may become clear during the joint planning process through a few suggestions from the patients. Most patients wanted a flexible therapy plan (see statement no. 2) that took their needs into account (see statement no. 3).

4.5.2 Support during therapy

Patients were also asked what they found un r supportive during therapy. A large number of patients felt it was important for therapists to show understanding (see statement no. 5). Being able to trust the therapist in the choice of therapy was considered just as important as discussions about their state of health (see statement no. 7). Many patients also found therapists with a sense of humour (see statement no. 14) to be supportive. The course of therapy should then be discussed together. During the exercises, many patients found it helpful when the purpose of the exercises was explained to them and when the exercises were suitable for everyday use (see statement no. 23) (ibid., p. 181ff).

4.5.3 Competence of therapists

Next, the respondents were asked about the competence of their therapist.

According to Dehn-Hindenberg (2008, p. 185f), patients did not primarily perceive the improvement of their symptoms and effective exercises as indicators of a competent therapist, but rather good communication and a high level of empathy. To illustrate this interesting result, the individual criteria are given the highest ratings in the following section.

A large number of respondents cited understanding their needs (85%) (see statement no. 21) and providing understandable explanations (83%) (see statement no. 24) as the most important criteria for the competence of therapists. In comparison, not quite as many patients considered effective exercises (80%) (see statement no. 22) and improvement in symptoms (73%) (see statement no. 25) to be the most important criteria for competence. The reason for this could also be that patients are perhaps unable to assess the effectiveness of the exercises in isolation (ibid.).

In addition, patients considered professional information (80%) (cf. statement no. 8-10) to be an important indicator of the competence of the therapists (ibid.). In a survey at the end of the therapy, patients were asked about their satisfaction with the information provided. This item was divided into information on treatment options, the effects of the disease and information on self-help (ibid., p. 200).

In addition, patients recognised the competence of the therapists in the successful organisation of the therapy (cf. statement no. 4) and in the nature and scope of the discussions (cf. statement no. 13) (ibid., p. 185f).

4.5.4 Motivation and working atmosphere

The therapeutic relationship is of central importance in motivating patients to undergo therapy. To this end, therapists must establish contact with patients and create an appropriate relationship of trust for the therapy. However, this expressly does not include an interest in private information that is not relevant to the therapy (ibid., p. 188f). For the therapy to be successful, the respondents needed a calm working atmosphere (cf. statement no. 26), clear instructions (cf. statement no. 24) and good guidance. The ability to listen (cf. statement no. 13) was also mentioned as a motivating factor (ibid., p. 188ff).

4.5.5 Expected behaviour of therapists

Patients also had the opportunity to write a free text. They were asked about their own influence and the influence of the therapist on the success of the therapy. The patients surveyed considered empathy (see statement no. 6) on the part of the therapists, the provision of information, explanations and advice (see statements nos. 8-10), followed by competence, effective exercises, diagnostics and monitoring (see statements nos. 22+23), the ability to motivate (see statement no. 15) and organise (see statement no. 4), as well as the friendliness (see statement no. 11), patience (see statement no. 16) and optimism (see statement no. 17) of the therapists (ibid., p. 192). Due to the fact that these were free-text responses and differentiating categories were formed during their analysis, no criterion was mentioned by more than 35% of respondents. However, as these criteria were nevertheless important, they have been included in the feedback form.

4.5.6 Therapy success

From the patients' point of view, although the therapists' soft skills, such as communication and empathy, are important for the therapy, the improvement of health, mobility and freedom from symptoms are the main factors contributing to its success (ibid., p. 196f). This means that although professional competence is essential for the success of the therapy, it is not evaluated, certainly also because laypeople are often unable to evaluate it.

Nevertheless, patients can assess whether the therapy has helped (Philippsen, 2007, p. 7). The success of the therapy is based on the professional skills of the therapist on the one hand and on the consideration of the needs described above on the other. In order to recognise the success of the therapy for patients, these aspects have been presented in statements 27 and 28.

Based on the assumption that satisfied patients can also be multipliers, as already described, this aspect was also added to statement no. 29.

When assessing whether patients are satisfied with the therapy, it should be critically noted that although they may have felt comfortable and rated the therapy as good, the therapy may still not have met professional standards and would have to be rated as poor from a professional point of view. This can happen, for example, if therapists interpret client-centredness in such a way that they avoid necessary, possibly painful exercises. In such cases, it would be more appropriate to explain the necessity of the measure and carry it out even if the patients feel uncomfortable.

4.5.7 Evaluation of the therapy provided

Finally, patients were asked to evaluate the therapy they received. Here, too, an endpoint-based, verbalised five-point scale was used. The highest rating was either *"very good"* [(1)] or *"yes, very good", and* the lowest *was "not good"* or *"no, not at all"* [(1)]. The following section describes only those criteria that have not yet been mentioned above and that were included in the feedback questionnaire created here because they were rated by at least 75% of respondents (the two highest ratings, 1 and 2, combined) (Dehn-Hindenberg, 2008, p. 255f).

Almost all respondents felt that they were treated with respect and accepted as human beings (see statement no. 12) (ibid.). As these criteria and the friendliness mentioned above are important in terms of customer orientation for service providers, they were included in the feedback questionnaire.

Of course, patient feedback must also be viewed as particularly subjective due to the personal involvement and dependence of the patients. Becker (2009, p. 220) states that it is precisely the subjectivity of the assessments that offers the opportunity for accurate interpretation. The soft skills that are difficult to measure and are asked about in the patient feedback questionnaire are particularly in need of this subjective interpretation.

4.7 Statements from the patient feedback questionnaire

Planning and organisation of therapy

The therapist...

1 ... involves me in the planning of therapy and then selects the right therapy method for me.

2. ... is flexible in planning the therapy.

3. ... takes my needs and wishes into account when selecting methods. wishes.

4. ... organises and plans the therapy in a meaningful way.

Communication and therapeutic relationship

The therapist...

5. ... shows understanding for my individual needs.

6. ... is compassionate.

7. ... talks to me about the course of therapy and my health problems.

8. ... advises me on therapeutic treatment options.

9. ...informs me about the effects of my illness on my everyday life.

10. ... informs me about self-help options.

11. ... always treats me in a friendly manner.

12. ... treats me with respect and accepts me as I am.

13. ... takes time to listen to me.

14. ... lightens the atmosphere with humour.

15. ... motivates me with encouragement and praise.

16. ... is patient when things don't work out.

17. ... shows optimism.

18. ... can accept my criticism.

19. ... identifies conflicts and problems and looks for the causes.

20. ... demonstrates a sense of responsibility when handling my data and medical history.

Guidance and therapy

The therapist...

21. ... recognises my needs during therapy and designs an individual treatment plan based on these needs.

22 ... selects effective exercises for me.

23. ... shows me exercises that I can use in my everyday life.

24. ... gives clear instructions that I can understand so that I know what to do and can do the exercises successfully.

25. ... achieve an improvement in my symptoms with the therapy.

26. ... conveys and ensures calmness and objectivity during therapy.

Result of the therapy

27 I feel better and can cope with everyday life more easily again.

28. When I come to the practice next time, I would like to be treated by the same therapist again.

29 I would recommend my therapist and the practice to friends and acquaintances.

4.8 The scale level of the feedback form

According to Becker (2009, p. 349), scales can be divided into qualitative and quantitative scales. Qualitative scales describe quality but do not classify it. They are nominal scales and, although they can be described as clear, they are not very comparable. Quantitative, i.e. numerical, scales can be used to determine mean values, standard deviations and other statistical values (ibid.). According to Becker (2009, p. 309), the scale level should be carefully considered. An odd number of levels to be assessed supports the tendency towards the middle, whereas with an even number of levels, the assessor must decide whether the performance shown is positive or negative, as there is no mean value. A large number of levels can overwhelm the feedback providers, as it requires a high degree of differentiation. In any case, the levels should be clearly anchored with corresponding values or words, as otherwise the subjectivity of the assessment increases due to the scope for interpretation of the levels (ibid.). Combined scales also allow for some, albeit less, scope for interpretation (ibid., p. 350). This refers to numerical scales that are additionally explained verbally. If there are several assessors, there may be differences in the interpretation of the numerical scale values (ibid., p. 351). By linking the numerical values verbally, this inaccuracy cannot be completely avoided through the interpretation of the values, but it can be reduced.

According to Schuler et al. (2003, p. 29), a behaviour-based rating scale, behaviour observation scale or behaviour ranking profile are suitable for 360° feedback. Behaviour observation scales represent several possible behaviours. The evaluators must then decide on a behaviour that has been demonstrated. Behaviour-based rating scales describe only one behaviour, which is then evaluated using a scale. A behaviour ranking profile evaluates an employee's suitability for this work (ibid.).

The feedback form developed here for patients is a behaviour-based rating with a multi-level verbal scale (Jung, 2011, p. 754). The behaviour to be assessed can be found in the statements in the questionnaire.

According to Porst (2014, p. 81), verbal scales have the advantage that respondents know exactly what is meant by the individual points and how they differ from one another. They do not have to think about the scale as much and do not make their own gradations. This makes the results of different assessors more comparable. Verbal scales are usually ordinal scales that specify a ranking of the possible answers (ibid.). In the case of the feedback form for patients, the ordinal scale consists of: *'Does not meet my expectations', 'Meets my expectations with reservations', 'Fully meets my expectations', 'Exceeds my expectations' and 'Exceeds my expectations to a high degree'.*

A 10-point Likert scale is used to evaluate behaviour, which is combined with the verbal scale mentioned above. While the verbal scale corresponds to a five-point scale, in which the grey-shaded middle range clearly indicates the rating required for a good assessment of the employee, those giving feedback must choose a number on the numerical scale. For example, the rating "The assessment *meets my expectations in full*" is assigned the numerical values five and six. The feedback providers must therefore decide whether this rating represents an upward trend or not (Benecke et al., 2014, p. 4f). The feedback providers' attention is drawn to this point by the grey background. In the next step, they should consciously question whether this criterion requires a higher rating. This is intended to prevent patients from giving too high a rating.

Edwards and Ewen (2000, p. 111f) point out that there should be an option to not answer. In this feedback form for patients, this is *provided* by the category *'Cannot* be *assessed'.* If this option of not answering is not available, feedback providers tend to give the average rating when they are uncertain (Edwards, Ewen, 2000, p. 157). Philipsen (2007, p. 78) notes that patients often give too high a rating due to social desirability, especially when there is no option to not answer. According to Porst (2014, p. 84), the assessment error 'tendency towards the middle' is reduced by the so-called escape point of non-response when assessors are uncertain or cannot or do not want to assess performance. If assessors now give a middle rating, this is also intentional. This increases the validity of the form. It remains to be seen to what extent the grey background colour of the average value in the feedback form for patients actually prevents them from giving the therapists too high a rating or manipulates them into believing that this answer is correct. To find this out, a test run with and without the grey background colour would have to be carried out. The results of these two runs could then be checked for high ratings and increased ratings in the grey area. To minimise errors, the individual categories were also described in the feedback form for patients.

Excerpt from the patient evaluation form:

Please rate each statement to indicate how your expectations were met.

Select the following rating	if ...
Not applicable	... you were unable to observe this statement
Does not meet my expectations	... you were not at all satisfied with the performance of this

	task. In your opinion, there is room for improvement here.
Meets my expectations with reservations	... you were partially satisfied with the performance of this task. Overall, you are satisfied with the performance of the tasks.
Fully meets my expectations	...you were **completely satisfied** with the performance of this task without any reservations
Exceeds my expectations	... You were **more than satisfied** with the performance of this task.
Exceeds my expectations	...you were particularly satisfied with the performance of this task. This is a **particular strength** of the therapist.

Please tick one box in each of these rating categories. Each category has two numbers assigned to it. You can now decide whether you would rate this category more positively or not.

Planning and organisation of therapy The therapist...	Can not be assessed	does not meet my expectations		meets my expectations with reservations		Fully meets my expectations		exceeds my expectations		Exceeds my expectations to a significant extent	
... involves me in the therapy planning and then selects the right therapy method for me	n.b.	1	2	3	4	5	6	7	8	9	10
							X				

The feedback form for patients is very detailed due to the 10-point Likert scale. A pre-test should be conducted to check whether patients are able to make these subtle distinctions. The associated five-point ordinal scale is certainly helpful in this regard. This allows patients to first decide on a category in the ordinal scale and then only have to choose the higher or lower number. The choice of words is critical. See 'Meets my expectations'. Patients certainly have different expectations of their therapists. Only a large amount of feedback can remedy this. Individual outliers can then be identified as such.

The statements in the 'Outcome of therapy' category should also be rated on a 10-point Likert scale combined with a five-digit verbal scale. The rating can range from *'not assessable'* to *'agree* 100%' to *'disagree completely'*. No area is shaded grey here, as the aim is not to focus on a specific range.

Excerpt from the evaluation form for patients:

	Result of therapy	Cannot be assessed	Completely disagree		Agrees 25%		50% true		75% true		100% true	
1.	I feel better and can cope with everyday life more easily again.	n.b.	1	2	3	4	5	6	7	8	9	10
2	When I come to the practice next time, I would like to be treated by the same therapist again.	n.b.	1	2	3	4	5	6	7	8	9	10
3	I would recommend my therapist and the practice to friends and acquaintances.	n.b.	1	2	3	4	5	6	7	8	9	10
	Result of therapy Total	n.a.	1	2	3	4	5	6	7	8	9	10
	Comments:											

The criteria are weighted equally by the scaling. This means that all criteria are assumed to be equally relevant for the evaluation of the therapist. It should be noted here that criteria that are interdependent are therefore underweighted (Becker, 2009, 194). Dehn-Hindenberg (2008, p. 256) established a correlation between the criterion *'therapeutic success'* and the criteria *'improvement of symptoms'*, *'empathy'* and *'acceptance as a person'*. *'Acceptance as a person'* could include both respect and friendliness. And although respect, friendliness and therapy success were considered important, as already mentioned in chapter 4.6, interestingly, according to Dehn-Hindenberg (2008, p. 264), they were of little significance to patients in their assessment of therapy success. Against this background, the above-mentioned correlation with *therapy success* can be disregarded.

CHAPTER 5

Guidelines for assessment

Rules and instructions on how to assess therapists are useful and necessary for the proper completion of feedback forms. They ensure transparency and better comparability of feedback forms by minimising errors in completion. However, they do not make assessments more objective (Becker, 2009, p. 214). Instructions describing the procedure for patients should be addressed to the respondents personally. An explanation of the purpose and use of the survey and a guarantee of anonymity are essential for honest answers. The estimated time required to complete the feedback form is just as important as clear instructions on how to complete it. At the end, respondents should be thanked for their cooperation and informed that they have actively contributed to improving the quality of therapy services (Bortz, Döring, 2006, p. 257). As the term "instructions" is somewhat cumbersome, it does not appear in the heading for patients. The heading of the instructions for patients is: Feedback on therapy. The instructions include a welcome and explanation of why the feedback is needed, an explanation of the scale and instructions on how to complete the form. The feedback form follows immediately afterwards in the same document. The font size is Arial 11 in the instructions with a line spacing of 1.15, and Arial 10 in the feedback form. The font size may be too small for older people, but a larger font would have made the form even longer. If necessary, the font size could be adjusted for older people.

5.1 Instructions for the 360° feedback (patients): Feedback on therapy

Dear patients

Your well-being is important to us. To ensure that you continue to receive the best possible therapy in the future, we ask you to evaluate your therapy and your therapist. Your feedback helps us to improve. That is why we use 360°

feedback for every employee in this practice. Our employees are regularly evaluated by their superiors, colleagues and patients. Employees can compare these assessments with their own, thereby identifying their strengths and weaknesses. Supervisors can then plan appropriate training courses to expand the skills of individual employees. Please take the time to rate the following skills of your therapist. Your information will be treated with the utmost **confidentiality**. The assessment will take approximately **15 minutes** to complete.

Instructions for completing the form:

Please enter the name of your therapist at the top. If you have had several therapists, e.g. due to substitutions, you are welcome to fill out a form for each one. These are available for you in the registration area.

In the following feedback form, you will find statements on planning and organisation, communication and therapeutic relationship, guidance and therapy, and the outcome of the therapy.

Please rate each statement according to how well your expectations were met.

See section 4.8, from page 52

Please place the completed form in the letterbox at reception or in the building's letterbox.

We thank you for your cooperation and hope you stay healthy. If you need to use our services again, we would be delighted to welcome you back to our practice at .
Your practice team.

5.2 Sample instructions for 360° feedback (self-assessment and peers)

The following instructions refer to a staff appraisal form that has been adapted and evaluated several times in study projects at the University of Applied Sciences and Arts in Hildesheim. Part A contains the employee's master data. Part B contains the staff appraisal according to the categories of specialist knowledge, skills, social competence and personal competence. Part C comprises the joint summary and the measures agreed upon.

Dear employees,

You have been asked by your line manager to complete a 360° feedback form. This will help you to develop your skills and make the best possible use of your resources. It will enable you to actively work on your professional development and present your own wishes and thoughts.

In addition, the feedback you provide on your colleagues gives you the opportunity to actively participate in quality improvement.

You have received assessment forms for self-assessment (pp. 1–12) and forms for assessing your colleagues (pp. 1–9). Your feedback on your colleagues will of course be treated anonymously. After the anonymous evaluation, you will receive a summary of the most important results of your assessment. These will be discussed with your supervisor in the subsequent evaluation meeting. In this meeting, goals and measures for the next assessment period will be jointly defined.

Please note the following information when completing the 360° feedback:

- The assessment forms (Part B) for self-assessment and for assessing your colleagues are identical. The instructions for both assessments are included in the feedback form for peers. Please complete parts A, B and C for your self-assessment. For the assessment of your colleagues, you only need parts A and B. On the cover sheet, you only need to enter your name and the name of the colleague you are assessing. Your name is for statistical purposes only. It will not appear in the evaluation.
- Please complete the assessment forms independently of each other.

- Please familiarise yourself with the criteria before starting the assessment. If you are completing the 360° feedback for the first time, you will need approximately 30 minutes for the assessment. The more familiar you become with the criteria, the easier and faster the feedback will be. Please allow yourself sufficient time before the assessment, free from distractions if possible, so that you can assess yourself and your colleagues appropriately and consistently.
- When assessing, please note that it is the current level of performance that is being evaluated, not potential. An assessment within the grey background or to the right of it means that there is no need for action in practice or on your part. If you are unable to comment on a criterion because you have not been able to observe it, for example, please select the category *"Not assessable"*.

  Once you have selected a category, please choose one of the two values on the 10-point scale.
- Please prepare for your evaluation meeting by reviewing the summary of the results you have received. In order to understand the assessment of the patients, you have received the patient feedback form. If you have also completed this form for yourself, you can compare the results of the summary with your own assessment.
- If your self-assessment has not been indicated in the evaluation, the summary of the values in Part C can help you to classify the results of the external assessments.
- Please record the contents of the discussion in Part C together with your supervisor.
- Based on the content of the discussion, the target agreements with possible measures for achieving these targets and the training plan will be jointly decided and recorded (p. 11).
- You will receive a copy of Part C: *Joint summary and measures*.
- Please allow approximately 60 minutes for your evaluation meeting.

Thank you very much for your cooperation!

5.3 Sample instructions for 360° feedback (supervisors)

Dear supervisor,

Please note the following information when conducting the 360° feedback:

- If you are conducting the assessments in paper form, please distribute the assessment forms for self-assessment and peer assessment to all participants. A copy in A3 brochure format has proven useful, as the explanations of the criteria are then directly next to the assessments. Each employee needs one copy for self-assessment and one for the assessment of their colleagues ( ). Please also distribute the blank feedback form for patients so that employees can understand how their feedback is evaluated and, if necessary, provide their own self-assessment.
- The full assessment form (parts A, B and C) is required for the assessment by supervisors and for self-assessment. Colleagues only need parts A and B to assess their peers.
- Please specify a time frame for completing the forms. This should not exceed two weeks after the assessment forms have been distributed. Please remind those involved to submit their forms on time.
- All participants should complete the assessment form independently of each other.
- Please ensure that the results are carried out and evaluated anonymously. An Excel table can be used for the evaluation.
- Please familiarise yourself with the criteria before the assessment.
- When assessing, please note that the current level of performance is being evaluated, not potential. An assessment within the grey background or to the right of it means that there is no need for action in practice. If you are unable to comment on a criterion because, for example, you were unable to observe it, please select the category *"not assessable"* or create a situation

in which the required assessment can be made. After selecting a category, please choose one of the two values on the 10-point scale.

- Once the evaluators have summarised the results, please arrange an appointment with each employee to discuss the results.
- Please prepare for each meeting and conduct it. You can use the instructions for the meeting provided here as a guide.
- If the supervisor's assessment has not been indicated in the evaluation, the summary of the values in Part C can help you to classify the results of the other assessments.
- Please record the contents of the discussion in Part C together with the employee.
- Based on the content of the discussion, the target agreements with possible measures for achieving these targets and the training plan are jointly decided and recorded.
- Employees receive a copy of Part C: *Joint summary and measures*.
- Sufficient time, free from interruptions, should be set aside for the evaluation meeting (approx. 60 minutes).

We wish you every success in the further development of your employees and your practice!

CHAPTER 6

Evaluation and summary of the 360° feedback assessment results

Feedback providers should know in advance who will have access to the results. Confidential handling of data and guaranteed anonymity are also beneficial for the honesty of the responses (Dietzsch, Kaschube, 2007, p. 8). This can be done by external consultants or coaches, who, however, make the process more expensive, apart from the time required for evaluation. External, trained coaches can, for example, use the individual results to identify when feedback providers have given a generally negative assessment, thereby distorting the overall result (Dietzsch, Kaschube, 2007, p. 16). Only by scientifically eliminating invalid responses, whether due to incorrect information or attempts at manipulation, can the result of the assessment be a collective evaluation of the employee's performance (Edwards, Ewen, 2000, p. 36).

The results should be summarised using software (Scherm, Sarges, 2002, p. 72) or password-protected online access. In recent years, the increasing use of technology in all areas has made the latter useful for completing questionnaires (Dietzsch, Kaschube, 2007, p. 10). The use of online access guarantees anonymity, keeps costs low and saves time (Werther, 2015, p. 2f). The results are stored on a server and evaluated immediately. Mean values and standard deviations can be calculated and deviations for self-assessment can be displayed (Dietzsch, Kaschube, 2007, p. 10). Not everyone is capable of interpreting the results, e.g. the significance of the standard deviation. Strongly deviating assessments of individuals would even have to be removed from the summary. It is questionable whether this can be done by laypeople.

There are now many providers on the internet. For a practice with five employees, this service can be offered for as little as £3,500 (plus VAT). The recurring costs of the evaluation are offset by the advantage of maximum data anonymity (Edwards, Ewen, 2000, p. 135).

If there are only a few evaluators, using a spreadsheet programme is a simple, quick and inexpensive alternative (Edwards, Ewen, 2000, p. 130), provided that the practice has the necessary methodological expertise in-house. However, in this case, it is questionable whether invalid responses will be eliminated scientifically, making it likely that the results will be distorted. The statistical evaluation of the results also requires certain knowledge of stochastics.

6.1 Documentation of results

The written summary of all feedback perspectives, which is handed out to the feedback recipient, should not be too long. It should refer to the most important differences in the assessments and be understandable for employees who are not trained in statistics. Weither (2015, p. 47f) notes that a 30-page results report does not automatically lead to more behavioural change. A graphical representation of the highest and lowest values with a profile overview by the different feedback groups and a comparison of the results with the self-assessment are important here (Scherm, Sarges, 2002, p. 51f).

According to Edwards and Ewen (2000, p. 142ff), there are profile reports, factor reports, perspective reports and comment reports. Profile reports give the average of all criterion assessments. The individual assessments of the self-assessment and the supervisor assessment are marked separately. The factor report shows the average of all criteria of a factor, i.e. a " " heading/category. The perspective report, on the other hand, shows the average of all assessor groups, i.e. the different perspectives. The commentary report reproduces the comments word for word (ibid.). Scherm and Sarges (2002, p. 68f) make it clear that the results report should contain both a graphical and a numerical representation of the data. Above all, the greatest similarities and differences between self-assessment and external assessment should be presented. The report is completed by an analysis of strengths and weaknesses and, if necessary, by requirement and target profiles. The reliability check must also identify major differences in criteria between individual feedback groups (ibid.). It is also essential that the highest and lowest ratings are clearly identifiable (Scherm, Sarges, 2002, p. 52). According to Edwards and Ewen (2000, p. 57f), external customers tend to give more positive ratings. This must be taken into account when interpreting the results of patient feedback forms.

In addition to the bar charts, managers should also receive a list of all individual assessments with the mean values and standard deviations. The standard deviations, which indicate the deviation from the mean value and can of course only be calculated from numerical values, should not be shown in the bar chart, as they would probably only confuse employees. The standard deviation should not exceed 1.0 for the criterion to be considered meaningful. This corresponds to the maximum deviation of 20% for less than 5% of feedback providers required by Edwards and Ewen (2000, p. 157). However, the standard deviation value of 1.0 only applies to the 10-point scale used here and would need to be adjusted for smaller scales.
Ratings below the desired value of five or six should appear in red in the summary, while values above eight, which can be considered strengths of the employee, should also be highlighted in colour, e.g. green, to indicate that they are " ". The latter only applies to the total values.

In the case of a small practice (fewer than four employees), supervisors should not receive the above table of all individual ratings, as they may be able to identify employees from the ratings. In this case, the evaluators should receive the additional information on the standard deviation, shown in the bar chart by the error bar.

6.2 Instructions for the 360° feedback (evaluators)

The Excel table used here can be requested from the author.

Dear evaluators,

please note the following information when evaluating the 360° feedback:

- Please ensure that the results are evaluated anonymously and do not disclose any information about your knowledge of the individual assessments.
- An Excel spreadsheet can be used for the evaluation. If an Excel spreadsheet cannot or should not be used, you can enter the sum of the individual ratings at the end of each category in the corresponding row of the feedback form.
- Assign an identification number to each feedback form. Use the initials of the employee, the

  evaluation group and a sequential number. Example: For patient feedback from John Smith, the identification numbers would be: JSS1, JSS2, etc. Enter the assigned identification number in the appropriate field on the paper form.
- The same applies to the feedback forms for equivalent employees. The identification numbers here are: MMG1, MMG2, etc.
- Please enter the values from the sheets in the corresponding column of the exit table. Delete the sample data first. If a criterion has been marked as 'not assessable', leave this field blank. Do NOT enter a 0 under any circumstances, as this would distort the average values in the table and thus the evaluation.
- Please note that some cells are locked to prevent accidental changes to the formulas. If you wish to change them deliberately, please enter the password: 360.

- If you require additional columns, you can expand the table accordingly. In this case, please check whether the corresponding columns are included in the automatic calculation.
- Please eliminate invalid responses. These are, for example, feedback forms that have given the same rating in all criteria. If a feedback recipient has rated between two numbers, enter the corresponding decimal number (e.g. 5.5).
- The data is automatically used to create bar charts showing the highest and lowest ratings and the average. These charts are summarised in the respective categories. They can be printed out and handed to the manager and the employee for the appraisal meeting. There are two different ways of displaying the charts; please check with the practice management to see which one should be used.
- Patient feedback: In addition to the bar charts, supervisors should also receive a list of all feedback with the mean values and standard deviations. The standard deviations are not shown in the bar chart, as they would probably only confuse employees. The standard deviation should not exceed 1.0 for the criterion to be considered meaningful. This only applies to the 10-point scale used here and would need to be adjusted for smaller scales.
- Ratings below the desired value of five or six are marked in red, while values above eight, which can be considered strengths of the employee, are marked in yellow. The latter only applies to the total values.
- Feedback from other perspectives: If it is a small practice (fewer than four employees), supervisors should not receive the above table of all ratings, as they may be able to identify employees based on the ratings. In this case, the evaluators should provide the additional information on the standard deviation.

Thank you very much for your support!

Your practice management

Example summary of patient feedback:

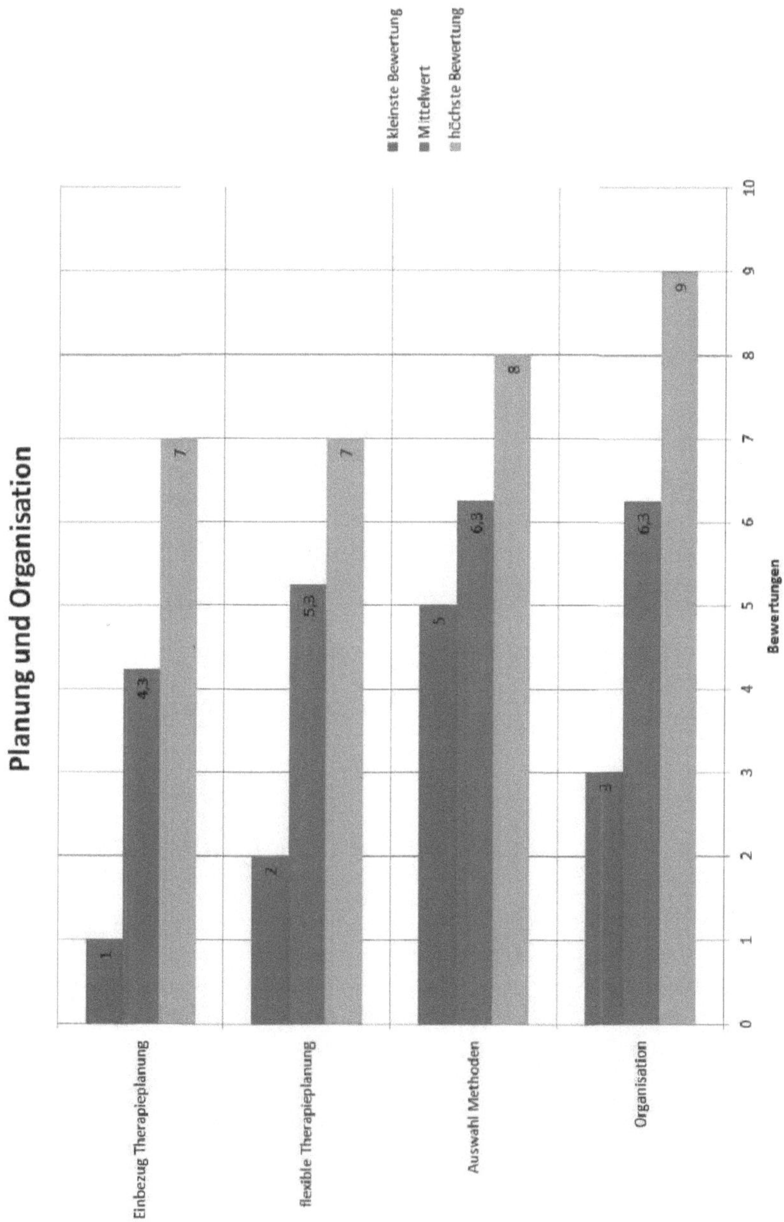

Example summary of peer feedback:

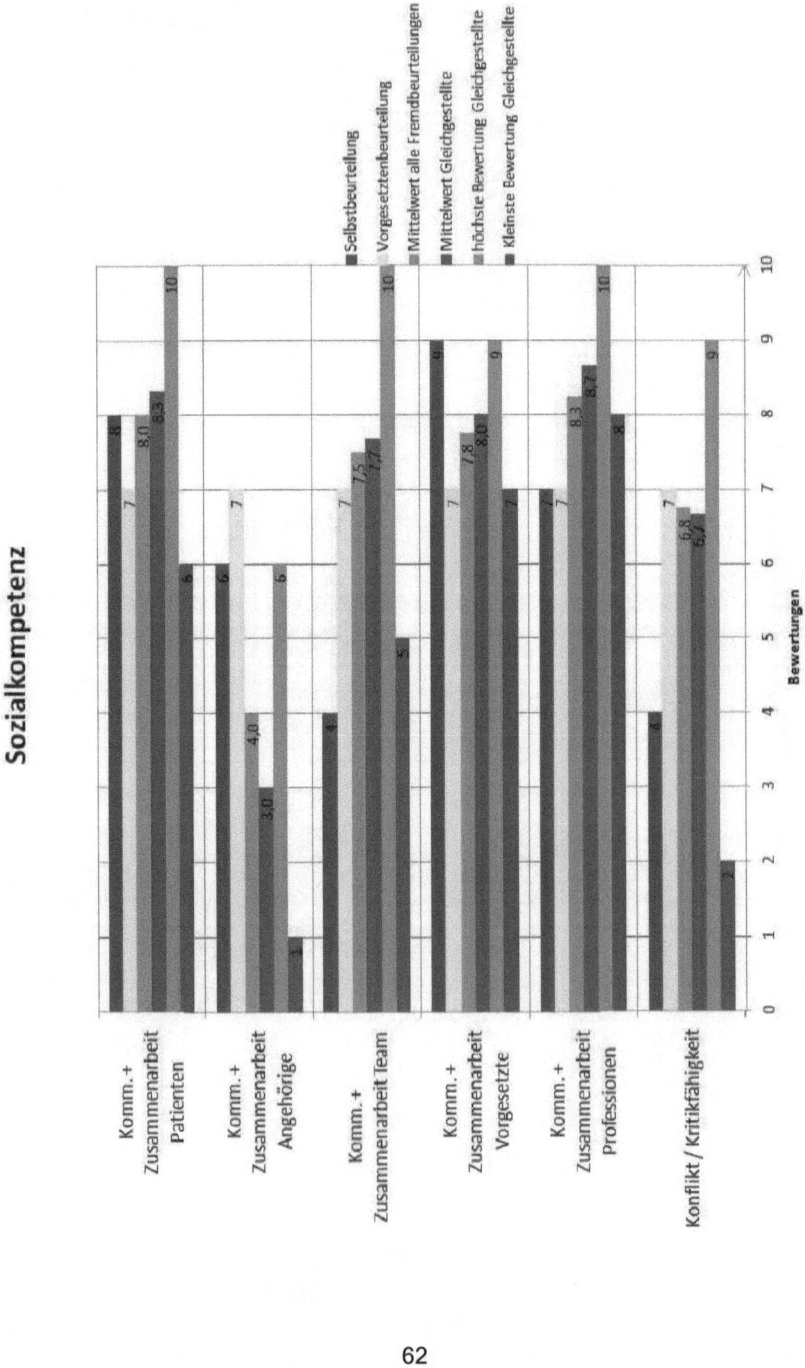

6.3 The evaluation meeting

Once feedback has been received from all perspectives and evaluated, a meeting with the employee is necessary. According to Section 82 of the Works Constitution Act, this is even the employee's right: the assessment of performance and opportunities for professional development should be discussed, and the employee should be given the opportunity to comment on planned measures. According to Scherm and Sarges (2002, p. 38), the feedback should be perceived as positive as possible by the recipient, as this increases acceptance of the feedback and the assessment. In addition to jointly formulating goals, employees should be offered support. Scherm and Sarges (2002, p. 42) state that there is a correlation between behavioural change after receiving feedback and the extent of support provided. Overall, a time slot of two hours should be scheduled for preparing for the meeting, the meeting itself, including verbal explanation of the feedback and the formulation of goals. Topics should also include tasks and functions as well as discrepancies between external and self-assessment. Supervisors should have the necessary communication skills for this. One option would be to hold the evaluation meeting together with colleagues. This would require a longer time frame of approximately three hours. In this case, it would be even more important for the supervisor to have psychological expertise in both conversation techniques and dealing with defensive attitudes. This option partially removes the anonymity of the survey (Scherm, Sarges, 2002, p. 52f). The discussion with employees should take place in an appreciative and pleasant atmosphere and should be as free from distractions as possible. Employees should be encouraged to engage in self-reflection (Scherm, Sarges, 2002, p. 56ff). According to Brenner (2014, p. 39), this can be achieved by asking open-ended questions, i.e. questions beginning with "What" or "How". The non-directive nature of these questions helps employees find their own solutions and explain the facts (ibid.). It is important to establish a connection to the employee's work during the conversation. Work situations can be addressed and analysed. If necessary, you can offer your own interpretations. To ensure that employees understand the main message of the conversation, it should not deal with trivial matters. However, a good mix of positive and negative feedback is helpful (Scherm, Sarges, 2002, p. 56ff). Brenner (2014, p. 33) also adds the need to communicate clearly and pay attention to the employee's signals during the conversation. This requires empathy on the part of the supervisor (ibid.).

The meeting should be divided into several phases. It begins with an opening greeting and an explanation of the purpose of the meeting and how it will proceed. This is followed by a review of the past assessment period, highlighting challenges, stresses and successes. The discussion of the individual results of the feedback should be limited to the strongest similarities and differences between the external and self-assessment and the feedback from patients. It is important here to highlight strengths and possible areas for improvement. If necessary, possible causes for discrepancies in assessments can also be analysed here. The next phase provides an outlook for the coming assessment period. The challenges and goals of the practice are identified, development needs and perspectives are discussed, and the goals of the employee and, if necessary, the need for further training are formulated together. At the end of the meeting, there should be appreciative feedback on the cooperation and a summary of the meeting with the results. Information should be provided about how the meeting will be documented and thanks should be expressed for attending (Alter, 2015, p. 46f). Conducting meetings with difficult feedback recipients requires special skills and approaches on the part of the supervisor. However, due to the scope of this topic, these cannot be explained here ( ).

6.4 Checklist for the conversation

Modified according to Alter, Urs (2015), p. 46f.

Preparation

Review the feedback from different perspectives and identify key points that should form the basis of the conversation.

- Arrange an appointment
- Find a time and place where you will not be disturbed
- Create a pleasant atmosphere (bright, attractive room, coffee, etc.)

Opening

- Welcome
- Ask how they are feeling
- Explain the purpose of the conversation and the procedure

Review of the previous assessment period

- Point out the challenges, stresses and successes in practice
- Highlight any goals achieved by the employee

Discuss the individual results of the feedback

- Point out the strongest similarities and differences between the external and self-assessment
- Review patient feedback
- Highlight strengths and potential areas for improvement
- If applicable, analyse possible causes for discrepancies

Outlook for the upcoming assessment period

- Identify challenges and goals for the practice
- Discuss development needs and prospects
- Jointly formulate the employee's goals and, if necessary, their training needs

Concluding the conversation

- Appreciative feedback on the collaboration
- Summary of the conversation with the results
- Inform about the documentation of the conversation
- Thank the other party for the conversation and end the conversation

CHAPTER 7

Conclusion

Although the introduction of 360° feedback in therapeutic practices involves costs and time, both the practices as businesses and the practice managers as entrepreneurs and employees can benefit from it. This book shows that it is possible to implement the system in a cost-effective manner. The costs of implementation and any necessary purchases are also tax-deductible and therefore do not have to be borne in full by the practices. It remains questionable whether practices can see the advantages presented here in relation to the high costs of 360° feedback. However, this book can help to change the attitude of practice managers towards 360° feedback.

Note: The assessment form and Excel tables mentioned in this book can be obtained from the author (r.benecke@web.de).

CHAPTER 8

Bibliography

Alter Urs (2015). Fundamentals of Communication for Managers. Wiesbaden: Springer Fachmedien Wiesbaden. DOI: 10.1007/978-3-658- 09273-3.

Barth Dieter (1999). Medical Marketing. From Advertising Ban to Patient Information: A Comparative Legal and Interdisciplinary Study on Communication between Patients and Doctors. Berlin, New York: Springer.

Beattie Paul F., Pinto Mary Beth, Nelson Martha K., Nelson Roger (2002). Patient Satisfaction With Outpatient Physical Therapy: Instrument Validation. In: PHYS THER 82 (6), pp. 557-565. Accessed on 07.11.2015 at: http://ptioumal.apta.orq/content/82/6Z557.full.

Becker Fred G. (2009). Fundamentals of Performance Appraisals in Organisations. Understanding and Principles of Performance, Appraisal Issues and Procedural Problems. 5th revised and updated edition. Stuttgart: Schäffer-PoescheL

Benecke Regina, Jungmann Anna, Kunert Mercedes, Wegener Romana (2014). 2nd evaluation of the personnel assessment form for occupational therapists in occupational therapy practices. Unpublished project report as part of the study project at the HAWK, University of Applied Sciences and Arts, Hildesheim. Winter semester 2014/2015.

Works Constitution Act (Betr.VG) in the version published on 25 September 2001 (BGBl. I p. 2518), last amended by Article 3(4) of the Act of 20 April 2013 (BGBl. I p. 868). Accessed on 04.12.2015 at: http://www.gesetze-im-internet.de/betrvg/ ______________________________ 82.html.

Works Constitution Act (BetrVG), Section 82, Employee's right to consultation and discussion (1) & (2). Accessed on 04.12.2015 at: http://www.qesetze-im-internet.de/betrvq/ 82.html

Betz Barbara (2014). Practice Management for Physiotherapists, Occupational Therapists and Speech Therapists. Berlin, Heidelberg: Springer Berlin Heidelberg. DOI: 10.1007/978-3-642-38407-3.

Bortz Jürgen, Döring Nicola (2006). Research Methods and Evaluation. Berlin, Heidelberg: Springer Berlin Heidelberg. DOI: 10.1007/978-3-540- 33306-7.

Brenner, Doris (2014). Conducting appraisal interviews with confidence. Wiesbaden: Springer Fachmedien Wiesbaden. DOI: 10.1007/978-3-658-

06999-5.

Bruhn, Manfred (2013). Quality Management for Services. Berlin, Heidelberg: Springer Berlin Heidelberg DOI: 10.1007/978-3-642-33992-9.

Dehn-Hindenberg, Andrea (2008). Patient Needs in Physiotherapy, Occupational Therapy and Speech Therapy. Idstein: Schulz-Kirchner.

Dietzsch-Kley Christina, Kaschube Jürgen. (2007). Study "Best Practice 360° Feedback": Current results and practical experience, [electronic resource] Accessed on 11 October 2015 at: http://www.hr-meter.com/files/uzkruz24.pdf.

Edwards Mark R., Ewen Ann J. (2000). 360° Assessment. Clearer feedback, higher motivation and more success for all employees. Munich: Beck WirtschaftsVerlag.

Flotho, Wiebke (2015). Client-centred approach. In: Steding-Albrecht, Ute; Jehn, Peter (eds). Occupational therapy: From treatment to action. Textbook for theoretical and practical training. 5th, unchanged edition. Stuttgart: Thieme. pp. 200–204

Gerpott Torsten J. (2013). 360° feedback process as a special variant of employee surveys. In: Domsch, Michel E.; Ladwig, Desiree (eds.), Handbook of Employee Surveys. 3rd edition. 2013. [electronic version]. Berlin, Heidelberg: Springer Gabler. pp. 127-162.

Jung Hans (2011). Human Resource Management. 9th, updated and revised edition. Munich: Oldenbourg.

Naidoo Jennie, Wills Jane (2003). Textbook of Health Promotion. Comprehensive and clear with many examples and projects from health promotion practice. Gamburg: Verlag für Gesundheitsförderung.

Nerdinger Friedemann W. (2014). Forms of assessment. In: Rosenstiel, Lutz von; Regnet, Erika; Domsch, Michel E. (eds.), Leadership of employees. Handbook for successful human resource management. 7th revised edition. Stuttgart: Schäffer-PoescheL pp. 201-212.

Parment Anders (2013). Generation Y. Wiesbaden: Gabler Verlag. DOI: 10.1007/978-3-8349-4622-5.

Lower Saxony Personnel Representation Act (NPersVG) in the version of 22 January 2007 (Nds.GVBL No. 2/2007 p. 11), last amended by Art. 3 of the Act of 30 June 2011 (Nds.GVBL No. 15/2011 p. 210). Accessed on 22 October 2015 at: http://www.schure.de/2047002/npersvg.htm.

Philipsen Tabea (2007). Investigations into patient satisfaction with medical care. Inaugural dissertation. University of Rostock. Accessed on 20 November 2015 at: http://rosdok.uni-rostock.de/resolve/id/rosdok_disshab_000000000097.

Porst Rolf (2014). Questionnaire. Wiesbaden: Springer Fachmedien Wiesbaden. DOI: 10.1007/978-3-658-02118-4.

Runde Bernd, Kirschbaum Dirk, Wübbelmann Klaus (2001). 360° feedback – tips for a best practice model. In: Journal of Work and Organisational Psychology A&O 45 (3), pp. 146–157. DOI: 10.1026//0932-4089.45.3.146.

Sausele-Bayer, Ines (2011). Personnel development as educational practice. Wiesbaden: VS Verlag für Sozialwissenschaften. DOI: 10.1007/978-3-531-94021-2.

Scherm Martin, Sarges Werner (2002): 360° Feedback. Göttingen: Hogrefe.

Schmacke Norbert (2005). How much medicine can humans tolerate? Bonn, Bad Homburg: KomPart-Verlagsgesellschaft.

Schuler Heinz, Hell Benedikt, Muck Peter, Becker Karlheinz, Diemand Andreas (2003): Science-Practice Forum. Design and testing of a multimodal performance assessment system: Individual module. In: Journal of Personnel Psychology 2 (1), pp. 29-39. DOI: 10.1026//1617- 6391.2.1.29.

Wahrig Gerhard, Wahrig-Burfeind Renate (1994). German Dictionary. With a lexicon of German language teaching. New edition. 1994. Munich: Bertelsmann Lexikon Verlag.

Werther Simon (2015). Introduction to Feedback Instruments in Organisations. Wiesbaden: Springer Fachmedien Wiesbaden. DOI: 10.1007/978-3-658-10497-9.

MIX
Papier | Fördert gute Waldnutzung
FSC® C083411

Kolibri 360 GmbH
Ferdinand-Jühlke-Straße 7
99095 Erfurt, Deutschland
produktsicherheit@kolibri360.de

Druck:
CPI Druckdienstleistungen GmbH
im Auftrag der
Kolibri 360 GmbH
Ferdinand-Jühlke-Str. 7
99095 Erfurt